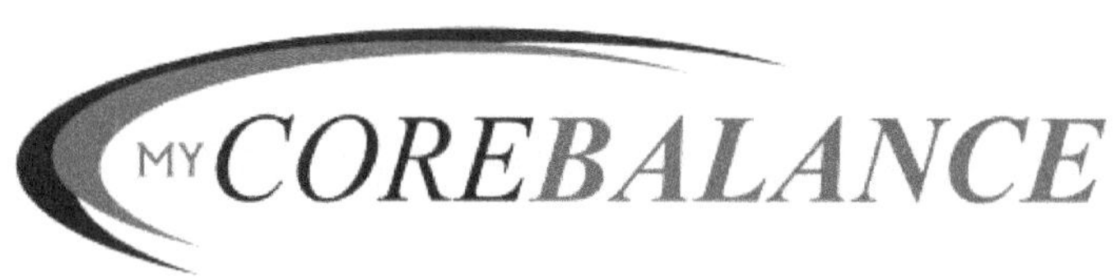

Fall

2019

Fitness Tracker

Chris Janke-Bueno

CONTENTS

WELCOME

Let's focus.

Hi,

Fall is a time to bring our energies in. It's a time for harvest, hopefully of your successful summer goals. But if your summer wasn't successful, and you find yourself more out of shape, just remember that fall is the time where you also get back on the routine. The summer travels are over, and it's time to get back to work on your health and fitness goals. We'll be checking in with this tracker periodically throughout the quarter. Use it as a helper, but not a crutch. Ultimately, let your body be the judge.

I'm excited to welcome you to the Fall 2019 Fitness Tracker. If this is your first experience at My Core Balance,

WELCOME!

Thank you again for your participation. I look forward to helping you **achieve your fitness goals... without injuring yourself.**

In health,

Chris JB

S.M.A.R.T. GOALS

Fall 2019

What do you *really* want?

What is your most important SPECIFIC goal?

How will you MEASURE that goal?

What ACTIONS will you consistently take?

Why? What's the REASON you want to achieve your goal?

How much TIME until you reach your big picture goal? Will it happen this quarter?

ASSESSMENT
Track your progress

Fall 2019

Start	**Goals**	**End**
Weight _________	Weight _________	Weight _________
Body Fat %	Body Fat %	Body Fat %
_________	_________	_________
Chest _________	Chest _________	Chest _________
Waist _________	Waist _________	Waist _________
Upper Arm _________	Upper Arm _________	Upper Arm _________
Lower Arm _________	Lower Arm _________	Lower Arm _________
Thigh _________	Thigh _________	Thigh _________
Calf _________	Calf _________	Calf _________
Neck _________	Neck _________	Neck _________

ASSESSMENT

Track your progress

	Start	End
How is your energy level?		
Stress level?		
How much back pain do you have?		
How are you sleeping?		

WEEKLY SPLIT
Your Workout Schedule

Your "split" refers to how you divide up your week. This is done from a macro level. No details yet. Ask yourself, "how do I want to divide my week?" Be sure to include stretching, core, strength, cardio, and rest. Take into account the other big obligations in your life: work, family, social, etc.

MON

TUE

WED

THU

FRI

SAT

SUN

NUTRITION

Your Daily Plan

Nutrition tracking has its place, but I've found that it can be more effective to create an "ideal day" and then work to try to reach that plan. Take a few minutes to write out what an ideal day looks like from a food perspective. If time, money, and eating out weren't issues, what's *your* perfect diet?
NOTE: you don't need to fill out all sections.

WAKE UP

BREAKFAST

SNACK

LUNCH

SNACK

DINNER

Fitness Education

Pyramid of Health

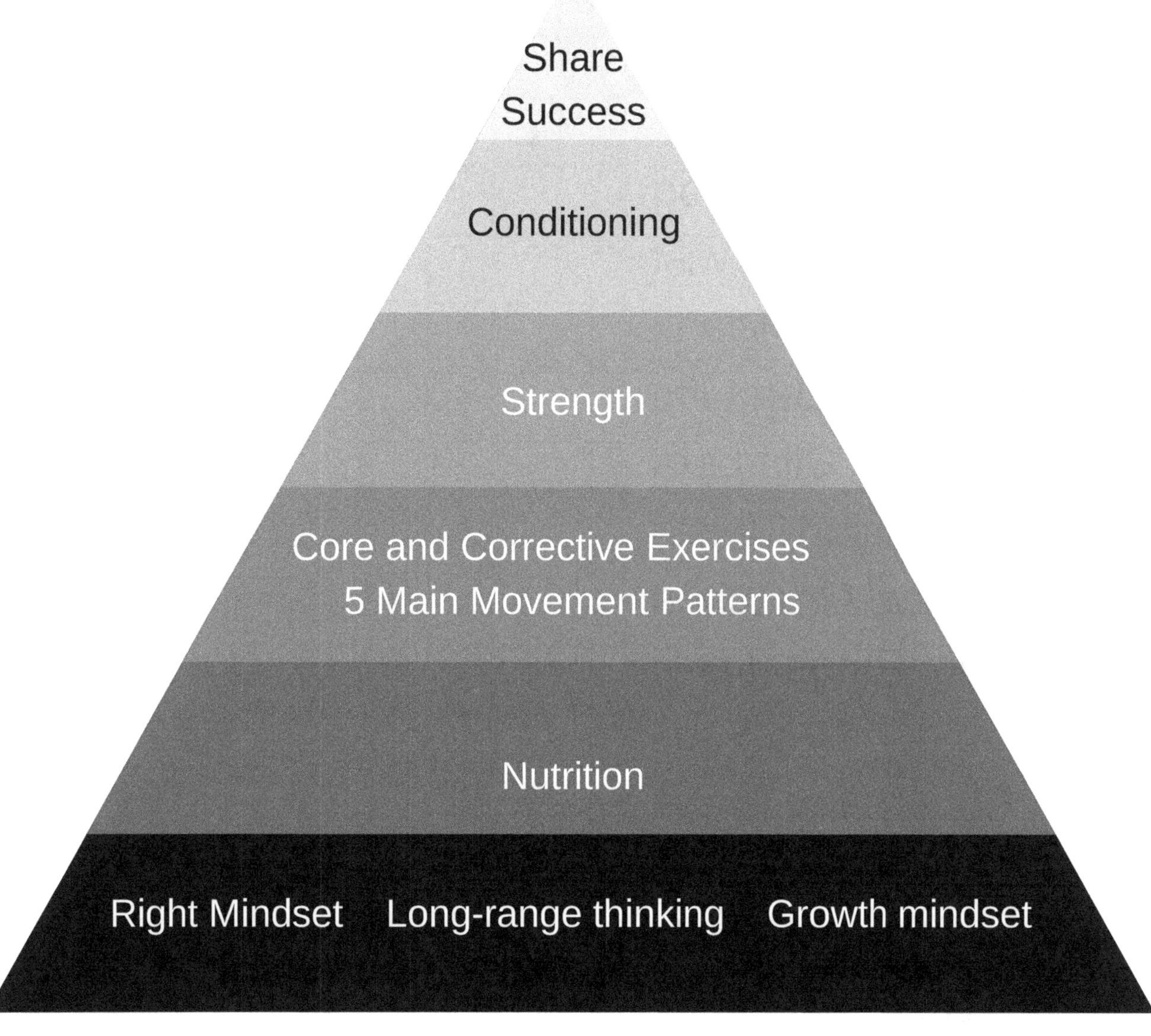

Workout #1

Dates

Donkey Kicks										
Supine Leg Raises										
Assisted Back Bridge										
Stand - Side Lateral Raise										
Standing Pullovers										
Bird-Dog										
Upper Spinal Floor Twist										
Push-Up to Side Plank										
Plank Alternating Leg Lifts										
Mountain Climbers										
Russian Twists										
Cross Crawl Crunches										
Hang From Rings (time)										
Bag Flips										
Incline Press										
Squat to Press										
Hammer Curls										
Tricep Kickback										

Workout #2

Dates

Quad Stretch										
Glute Bridges										
Knee Extensions										
Lucky Pennies										
Static Wall										
Static Wall Crossover										
Cats and Dogs										
Full Sit-Ups										
Bear Crawl										
Crab Walk										
Pistol Prep 1 Hand Down										
Inchworm										
Assisted Pistol Squat										
Bench Press										
Cable Row										
Jump Squat										
Rubber Band Push Ups										
Tricep Pushdown										

Workout #3

Fall 2019

Dates											
Quad Stretch											
Pigeon Stretch											
Foot Circles											
Runner's Stretch											
Counter Stretch											
Chest Stretch											
Rear Deltoid Stretch											
Side Arm Circles											
Hip Crossover											
Upper Spinal Floor Twist											
Cats and Dogs											
Bird-Dog											
Cross Crawl Crunches											
Inchworm											
Squat											
Bench											
Bent Over Row											
Superman											

Workout #4

	Dates									
1-Leg Glute Bridge										
Flutter Kicks										
Outer Thigh										
Inner Thigh										
Crunch Position Leg Raise										
Straight Leg Walk										
High Knee Walk										
Stranding Hamstring Curls										
Windmill										
Standing Hip Flexor Stretch										
Walk Outs										
Table Top to L Sit										
H & K - Arm Circles										
Speed Skaters										
1-Arm Row										
Battle Ropes										
Jacob's Ladder										
Hallway Side Shuffle										

Workout #5

Dates

Glute Bridges											
Hip Crossover											
Cats and Dogs											
Straight Leg Ab Engage											
Back Plank											
Plank Side Leg Taps											
Front Plank Twist Up											
Downward Dog											
Static 90 Alt. Crunches											
Superman											
Static V or Full Sit-Up											
Circle Crunches											
Inchworm											
Bear Crawl											
Core Roll											
Jackknife											
Knee-Ins											
Twisties											

Workout #6

Fall 2019

Dates

Bridge with Strap											
90-90 with Ring											
Hip Lift											
Hip Twist											
Cats and Dogs											
Side Arm Circles											
SF Elbow Curls											
SF Goal Posts											
SF Wall Glides											
Inchworm											
Glute-Ham Machine											
Squat											
Overhead Press											
Dead Lift											
Barbell Curls											
Hanging Leg Raises											
Weighted Windmill											
Overhead Tri Extension											

Cardio

H.I.I.T. and L.I.S.S.

Dates

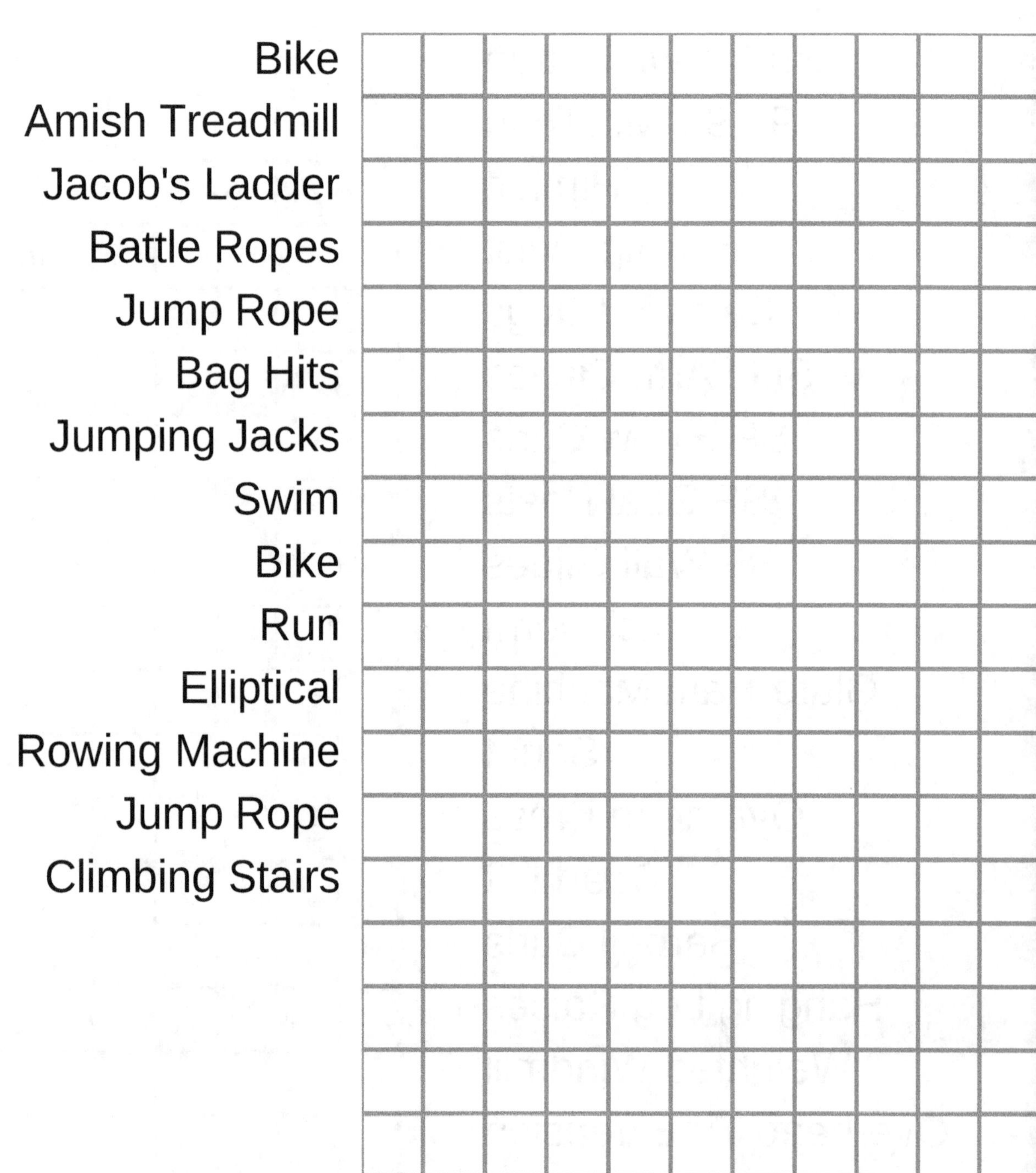

Bike										
Amish Treadmill										
Jacob's Ladder										
Battle Ropes										
Jump Rope										
Bag Hits										
Jumping Jacks										
Swim										
Bike										
Run										
Elliptical										
Rowing Machine										
Jump Rope										
Climbing Stairs										

H - high intensity   L - low intensity

Evaluation
How did you do?

What worked well?

What didn't work well? How will you change it?

Did you reach your goal? Why or why not?

NOTES

NOTES

To purchase the next fitness tracker book, *Winter 2020*, visit
www.mycorebalance.com